serious health issues. She's always been very comfortable in her own skin, with no image problems and mostly very happy. But, she has also never had any doubts about her disinterest in sports or competition of any kind. Looking back, we now realize that over time we had been conditioned to accept Abbie's inactive lifestyle as just a large part of her personality. Our mistake.

The truth is the experts are right about effective exercise for children. It can be as little as sixty minutes per day and it can be as easy as walking. You, the parent or guardian, must simply take charge, be committed to helping your child find some form of fun and effective exercise and find the time! In our case, Abbie and I usually choose to go to bed an hour earlier each night and get up an hour earlier each morning...sometimes as early as five am. That might sound extreme, but we actually look forward to those early morning walks when it is just the two of us, hand in hand, in the dark and under the stars. This is not just our time to exercise together, but also our 'daddy-daughter' time each day. Not only have we both become much fitter in the process, but our relationship has been changed forever! This journey has truly been a win-win for us.

We have no doubt that, had we not intervened when we did, Abbie's fitness level would have continued to deteriorate. Instead, Abbie, now thirteen years old, has become a very fit girl with a great attitude towards wellness. Although still not overly active, Abbie has developed a very healthy respect for the need to exercise and eat right every day... a respect that we are confident will serve her well for a lifetime. It is our sincere wish that this book will help you and your child get on the road to your own 'Get Fit' story.

Yours in fitness,

Doug Werner

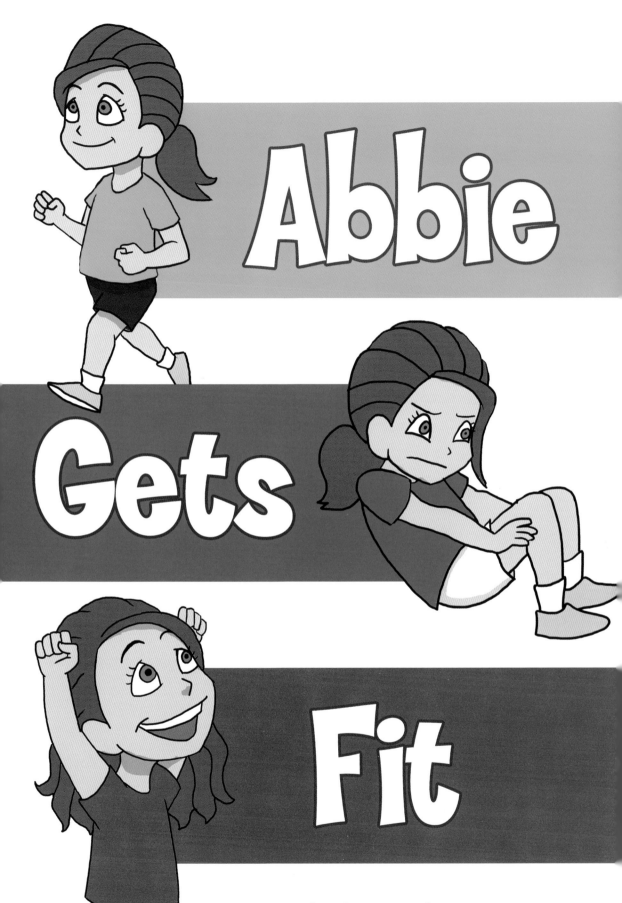

Abbie Gets Fit

By Doug Werner

illustrated by Rafael D. Nazario

"Daddy, Daddy, Daddy… look, I had my fitness test in school today."
Nine-year-old Abbie rushed to greet her Daddy at the door, with
her curly brown hair bouncing along behind her. She jumped into
his arms and handed her test score to him. "Look at my scores
Daddy…did I do good?" she asked, as he carried her across the
room. "So, Abbie, tell me all about it," her daddy said as they sat
down together in his favorite big blue chair.

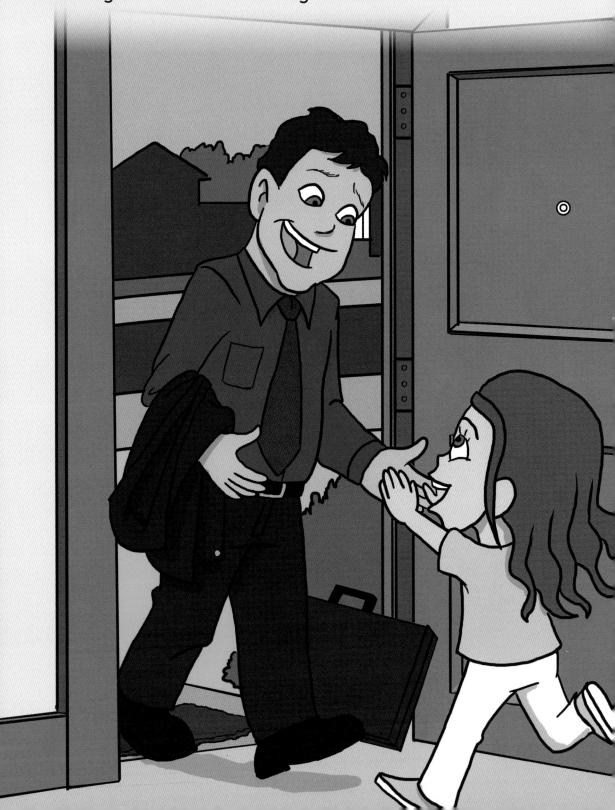

Abbie sat up proudly in her daddy's lap, "Well, first we had to run four laps around the soccer field while Ms. Hatch timed us with a stop watch. Daddy, that was really hard," her bright blue eyes lit up as she nodded her head. "Why was it so hard, Abbie?" he asked. "Daddy, I tried to keep up with everyone else, but my legs got real tired and I couldn't breathe very well," she explained while rubbing her thighs with her hands.

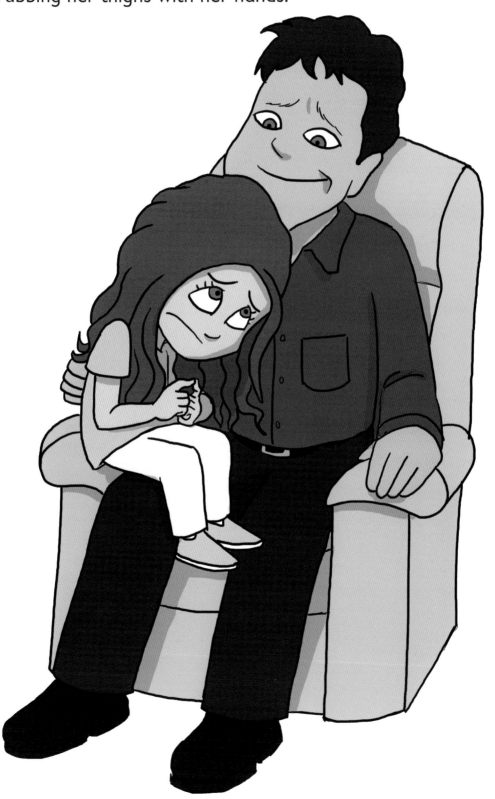

"I'm sorry, Abbie, so how long did it take you to run the four laps?" he asked. "Look, Daddy, it's right here on the paper," she pointed to the report.

He read it, "It says it took you twelve minutes and thirteen seconds to finish. Is that right?" "Uh, huh," she nodded. "Is that good, Daddy?" she asked with a big toothy grin.

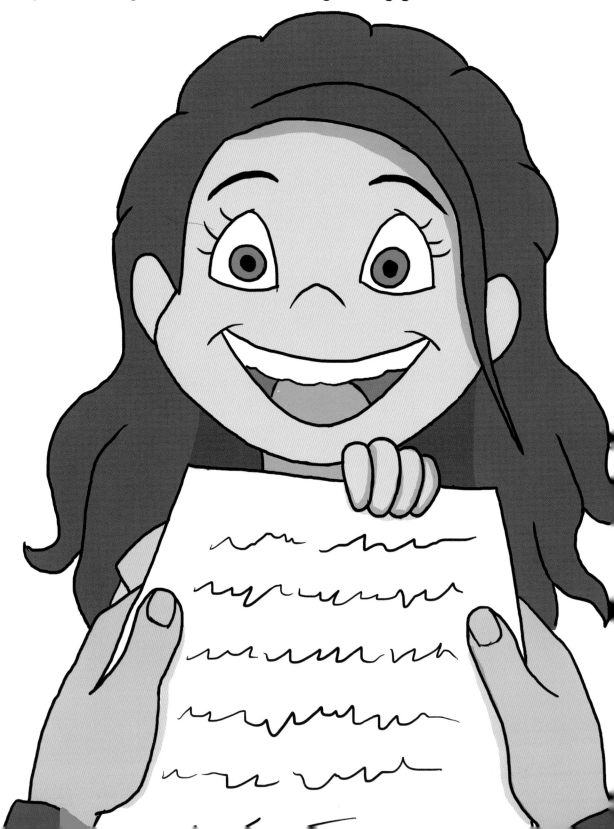

"Well, the report says that your goal was eleven minutes, so you missed by over a minute. What do you think, is that good?" he asked while handing the report back to her. Abbie lowered her head and pouted, "No, I guess not, huh, Daddy?" He smiled and put his hand on her shoulder, "It's not too bad, but I know that you can do much better. Do you think that you can do better than that, Abbie?" he asked. She paused for a second and then replied, "I think I can, Daddy, but how do I get better?" He smiled and said, "Well, I can help you, Abbie, but first, tell me about the rest of the test."

"Well, next we went into the gym to do curl-ups," she explained, "and I did eight." Abbie jumped down on the floor and showed her daddy how to do a curl-up. "Like this, Daddy," she said. Lying on her back, with her feet flat on the floor, her knees up and hands resting near her hips, she 'curled up' her stomach muscles and slowly raised her shoulders off the floor several times.

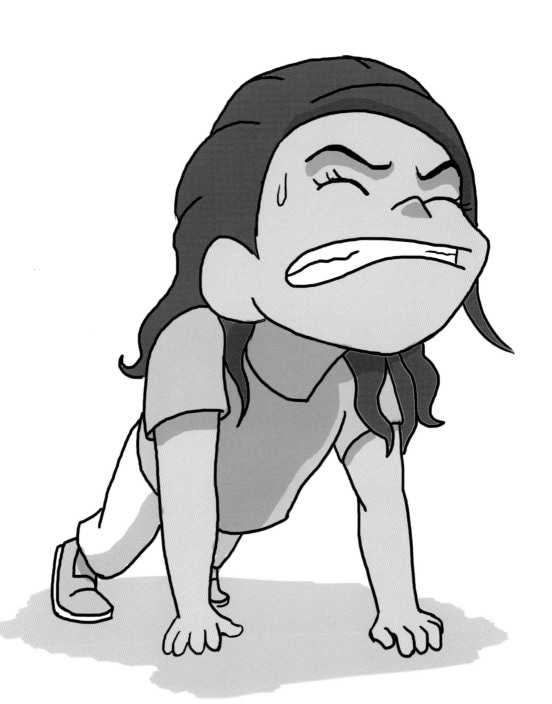

"That looks very good, Abbie, but was eight curl-ups enough?" he asked.

She frowned and lowered her head, "No, we were supposed to do twenty," she answered, "but I did try to do more." Then she shrugged, "You know, Daddy, curl-ups are really hard to do." He leaned over and kissed the top of her curly head, "Okay, I'm sure you tried hard, Pumpkin. What did you do after the curl-ups?" he asked, glancing back at the report.

"Next we did push-ups, like this," Abbie demonstrated a push-up at his feet. While lying on her stomach, with her hands flat on the floor near her chest and her back straight, Abbie pushed herself up and down off the floor with her arms. "Those are hard too, Daddy, but I did ten of those," she gasped after a couple of push-ups. "Okay, well that's better. What did your teacher have to say about that?" he asked.

"Well, Ms. Hatch said that if we did fifteen push-ups and twenty curl-ups, and ran the mile in eleven minutes, we could write our name up on the wall chart," she explained. "Oh, and Daddy, Charlotte and Hannah got to put their names up on the wall," she grinned. Her daddy smiled. "That's great, Abbie, they must be very happy." "Yes, they are. Hannah wrote her name in pink and Charlotte used purple; it was so pretty. They're so lucky, Daddy." Then she frowned, "I wish I could put my name on the wall too…I'd use a blue marker," she cheered while jumping into her daddy's lap again. "Did I do good, Daddy, did I?" she pleaded.

Her daddy sighed, placed the report on the side table and wrapped both arms around his little girl. "Well, Abbie, you did okay, but we both know that you can do better, right?" he asked, looking straight into her eyes. "Yes, Daddy, but will you help me?" she sighed and laid her head on his shoulder. "Yes I will, Abbie, I'd love to help you," he answered, "but, you have to promise me that you will try very hard, and that you will exercise every day. No excuses, okay?"

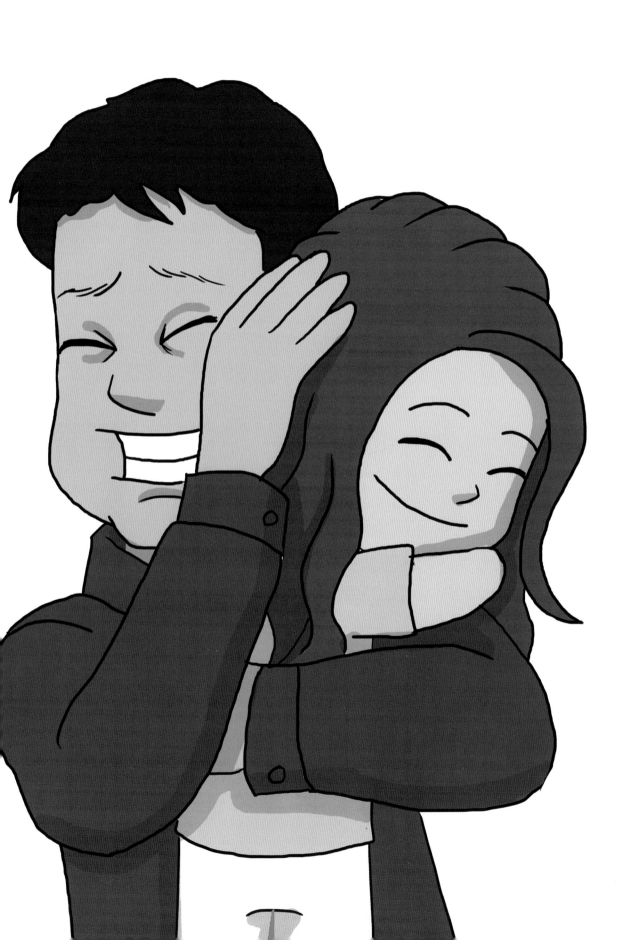

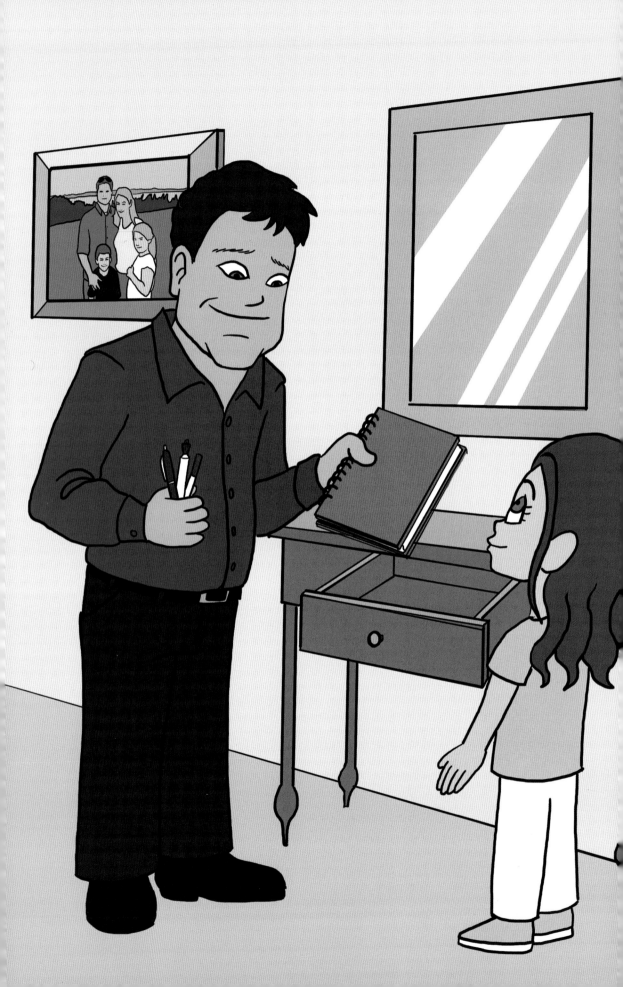

Abbie looked up at her daddy, smiled, and nodded her head. "Okay, Daddy, okay. I do want to get fit and I'll try really hard and I'll exercise every day. When can we start, Daddy?"

"We can start tomorrow, Abbie, but first let's make a workout chart and set some goals for you, okay?" He pulled out a notebook and pen. "Okay Daddy," Abbie answered, "but, what are goals?" Her Daddy explained that goals are like wishes… anytime you wish for something; you're actually setting a goal for yourself. The stronger the wish, the better the goal.

"Abbie, you just told me that you wished you could put your name on the wall chart, right?" he asked. She answered him with a big smile, "Yes, and I'd use a big blue marker Daddy!"

"Okay, so that's a very good goal for you. It's something that you're really excited about, and it's also something that we both know you can do… right?" he asked. "Oh yes, lots of other kids can do it, so I know I can too."

"Great! It's important that you believe in your goals and that you're really determined to achieve them, so let's write that goal at the very top of your workout chart." In bold capital letters he wrote on her chart… PUT MY NAME ON THE WALL! "Now, tell me Abbie, what will you need to do to reach that goal?"

Abbie looked at the report. Her next fitness test would be in the spring and the goals would be even higher. "Wow Daddy, it says that I will need to run the mile in ten minutes and thirty seconds, do thirty curl ups and twenty push-ups." He smiled, "That's okay, Abbie, I'm sure you can do it, but you'll have to work hard and stay focused on your goals. So, let's put those goals on your workout chart too." He wrote the goals across the top of the chart and then looked at her, "Now, what are some other good goals for you, Abbie?"

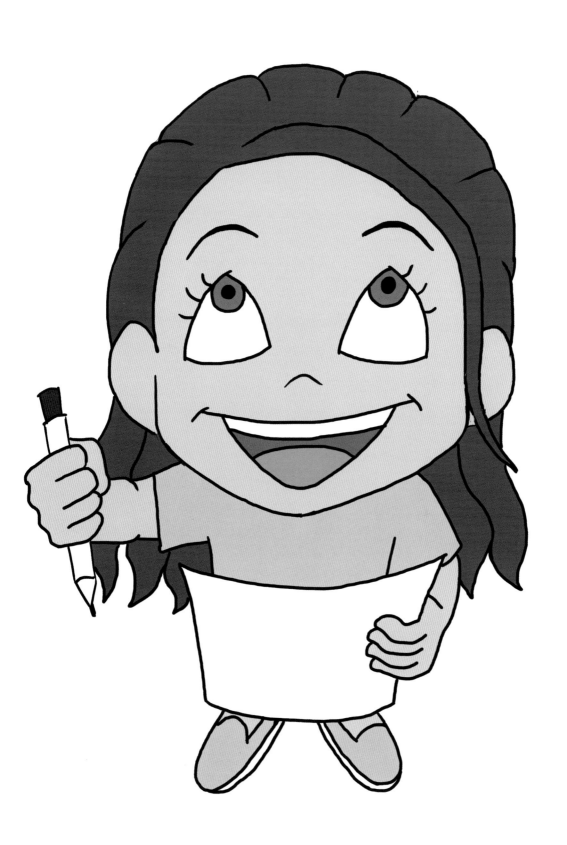

"Well Daddy, I wish that I could wear the kind of clothes my friends wear. Will exercise help me do that?" she grinned. "Of course it will, Abbie, exercise will help make you fitter. And if you're fit, you'll look better in all types of clothes," he answered. "Yay, and if I'm fit, will I be able to play games better too?" she asked.

"Oh yes, when you're fit you'll have more energy for lots of things, including homework and chores too," he winked at her. "There are many very good reasons to get fit Abbie, so let's review your goals and get ready to start, okay?" her Daddy gave her a big high five.

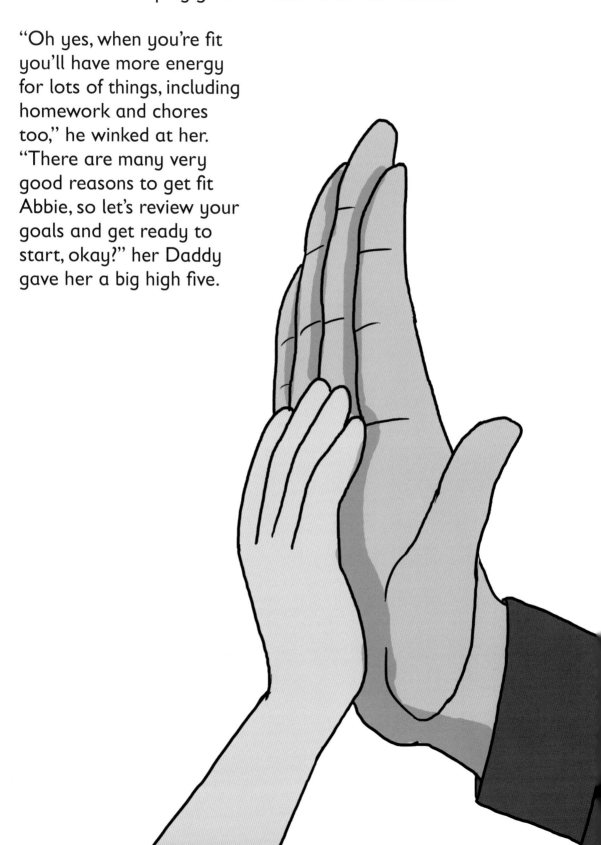

Abbie's next fitness test was nearly six months away. To pass the test and get her name on the wall, she would have to get much fitter. She had a lot of work to do, but her daddy knew she could do it if they stayed focused on her goals, started slow, and gradually increased her exercise level every day. They sat down and looked at all of the goals on the chart. Abbie agreed that she would exercise every day and she put her initials next to each goal. She then handed the chart back to her daddy, smiled and said, "Okay Daddy, I'm ready to go. When do we start?"

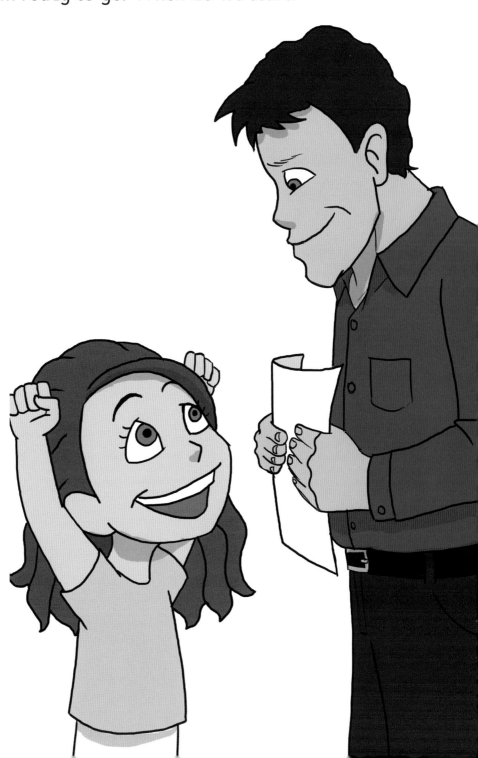

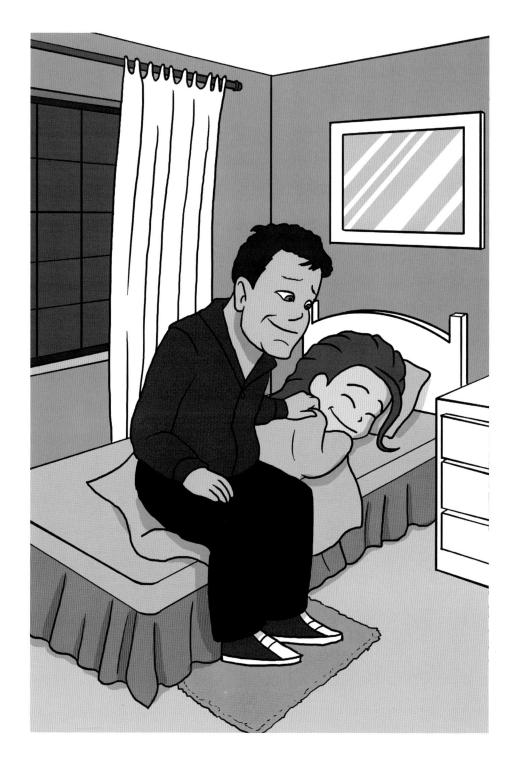

The next morning, while the rest of the family still slept and the sky was still dark, Abbie's daddy quietly tip-toed into her room and gently rocked her shoulder. "Abbie, time to get up," he whispered in her ear. She moaned, struggled to open her eyes and winced at him. "Daddy, what time is it?" she yawned. "It's time to exercise, Honey," he answered, "we are going to start every school day with a nice walk together. So it's time for you to wake up and let's get going."

She rolled over in bed and pulled the blanket up under her chin. "Oh, Daddy, do we have to?" He turned on the light. In his hand he had her workout chart with her fitness goals and her initials on it. He sat next to her, put his hand on her shoulder and looked into her sleepy eyes, "Abbie, do you remember what we talked about yesterday? These goals are very important to you. We're doing this for you. If you don't want this bad enough, it will never happen. It's up to you Honey, do you want to get fit? Do you want to get your name up on that wall?"

She thought about it for a moment and then suddenly sat up! "Oh yes Daddy, I want to get fit and I want to get my name up on that wall. Let's go!" she cheered as she jumped out of bed.

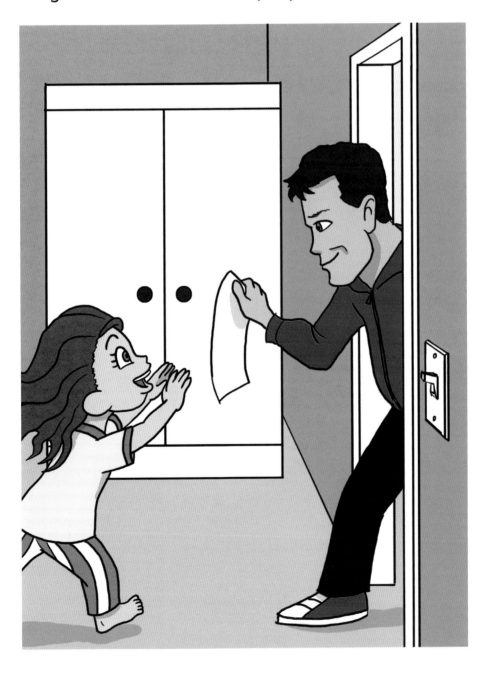

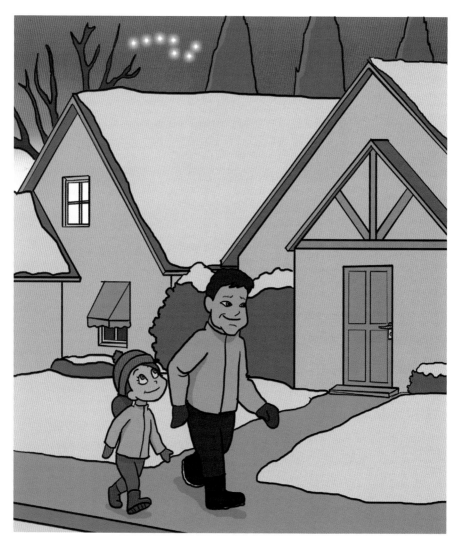

Abbie and her daddy walked together nearly every day for six months. At first, Abbie struggled a little and they would only walk for fifteen or twenty minutes. As she got used to it and started becoming more fit, Abbie and her daddy gradually added time each day until eventually they were walking for one full hour. While they walked, always hand in hand, they would talk and play word games. Some mornings they would see deer running through their neighborhood and occasionally they would see a shooting star. Abbie loved gazing at all of the stars in the early morning sky and she became very good at finding the Big and Little Dipper. Sometimes while they walked, Abbie would just talk about her friends and school, and other times her daddy would test her spelling, her math, or her geography. Not only was Abbie getting fit, but her grades in school started to improve and she and her daddy were getting to know each other much better. They both began to really look forward to their daily walk together. They walked morning, noon or night. They walked when it was warm and they walked when it was cold.

They walked in the rain and they walked in knee-deep snow. Nothing could keep Abbie and her daddy from their daily walks. Over a very short time, Abbie's fitness level, her grades and her relationship with her daddy improved a lot… and he was getting fitter too. Each night, just before she went to bed, Abbie would alternate doing her curl-ups and her push-ups. She started with five of each, while her daddy made sure that she did each one perfectly. Gradually, she did more curl-ups and push-ups, until just a few months later she could do over twenty push-ups and over one hundred curl-ups! Abbie proudly marked her workout chart with those numbers everyday. Her fitness level improved daily and with it, so did her self-esteem and confidence. One night, feeling proud and strong, Abbie decided she wanted to see exactly how many curl ups she could do without stopping. She stunned her whole family when she managed to do a whopping two-hundred curl ups! A very long way from the eight she had done on her first fitness test!

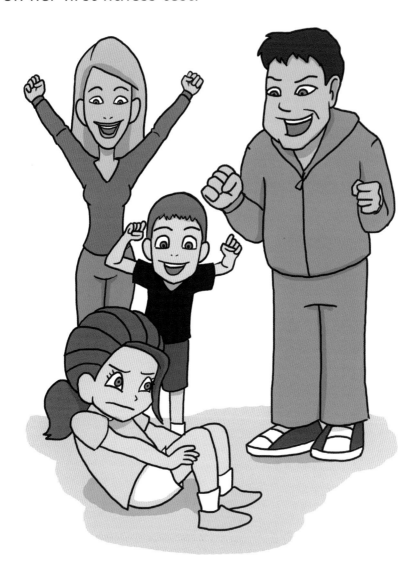

About two months before her fitness test, Abbie and her daddy began to jog at the end of their walk. At first, they only jogged one block. This was harder for Abbie, but her Daddy taught her to keep her head up and shoulders back while she ran, which made it easier. She learned to keep her upper body relaxed, hands swinging gently by her side, with her feet low to the ground, pushing off on her toes and landing on her heels. Over time, Abbie began to enjoy the jogging and she increased her distance gradually one block at a time. By the end of the six months, she was jogging one full mile with very little difficulty.

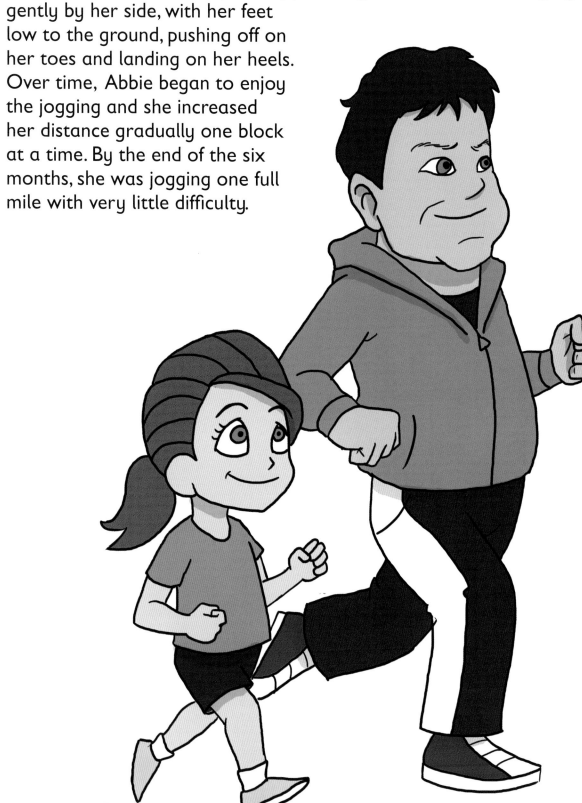

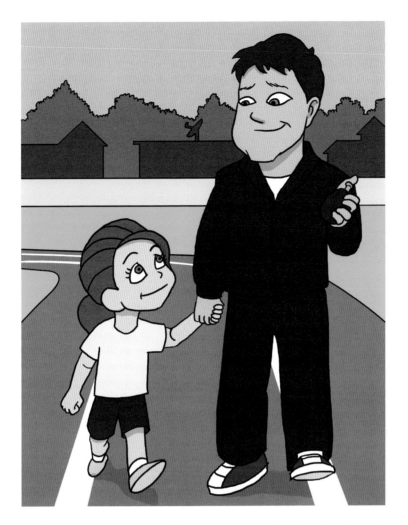

One week before the spring fitness test, Abbie's daddy took her to the school to do a practice mile on the track. He brought a stopwatch and helped her warm up. "Abbie, we're going to run four laps together and I'm going to time us with this watch. But don't worry, I won't go too fast. You need to stay with me every step of the way and keep thinking about your name on that wall…okay?" Abbie swallowed hard, cracked a smile and nodded, "Okay, Daddy," she said. He put his hands on her shoulders and said, "Look Abbie, your legs might start to get heavy and it might be harder to breathe after a while, but that is very natural and it won't hurt you…so don't let that slow you down. Keep reminding yourself of that goal and remember that it's only one mile…it will be over soon and daddy will be there every step of the way. I know you can do this and so do you…right?"

She looked up at him, smiled and nodded again, "Yes, Daddy, I can do it!" "Great, don't forget that. You can do this Abbie!" He gave her a big hug and they lined up on the track next to each other ready to go.

They started their run with a light jog side by side, using the running technique that he had taught her. "You're doing great, Abbie; keep your head up, breathe deep, and relax. We'll be done before you know it," her daddy said as he cheered her on. The girl who could barely finish a mile six months earlier was suddenly starting to look like a real runner.

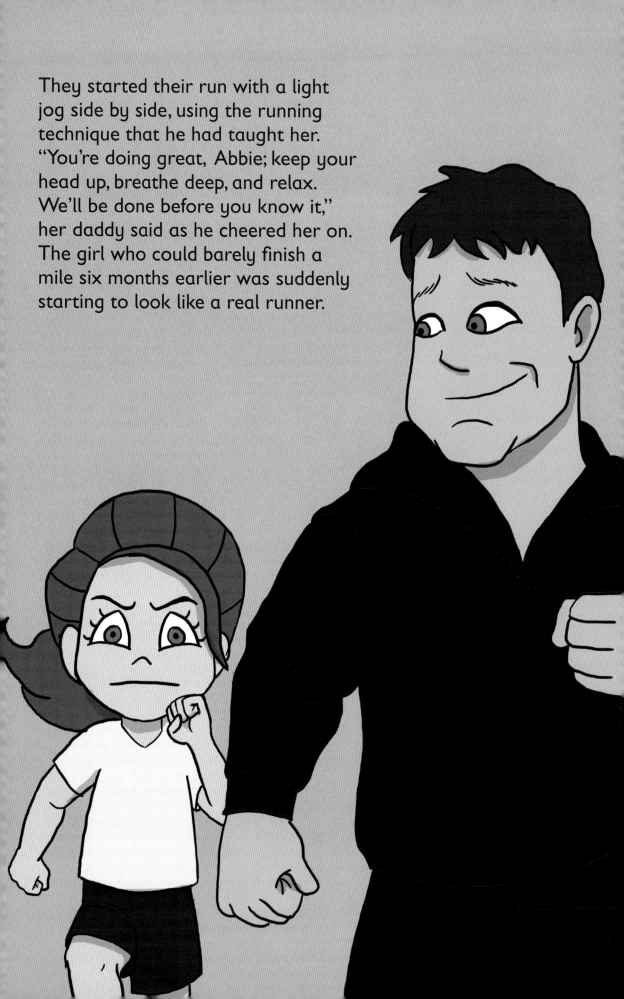

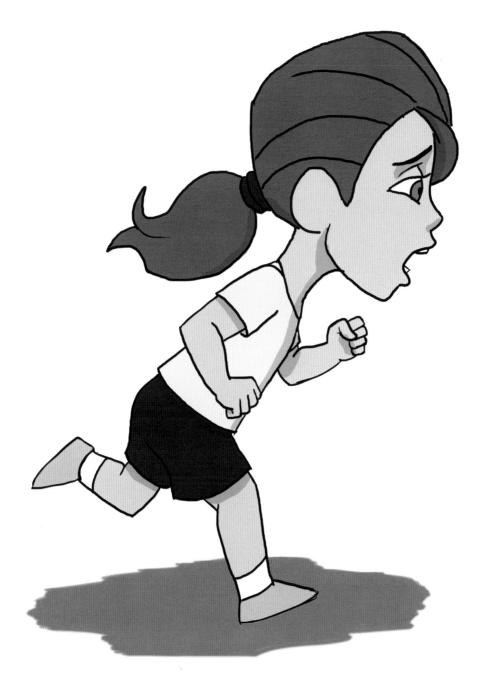

After each lap, her daddy would read off the time from the stopwatch. They did the first lap in nearly two minutes and Abbie felt good. They did the second lap in about two minutes too, but she started to breathe more heavily.

Gradually, her legs began to get tired, she slowed down a little bit and it took two and a half minutes to finish the third lap. As they started the final lap, Abbie was getting very tired. She complained about the burning in her lungs and tired legs. She had never run this fast for so long and she wanted to slow down, but her daddy kept nudging her on. "Come on, Abbie, this is the last lap. We'll be done soon. Don't stop now, you can do this!" he urged while keeping the pace.

Abbie's daddy knew that although the 'health goal' for her fitness test was ten minutes and thirty seconds, the 'challenge goal', for only the fittest kids was nine minutes and fifteen seconds! He now realized that not only could Abbie beat that time, but with a little extra effort she could actually beat eight minutes, which would be a very big improvement from her first test.

As they approached the halfway point of the last lap, her daddy turned to her and said, "Abbie, how bad do you want your name on that wall?" "Real bad, Daddy, real bad," she panted. "Okay then, Abbie, let's go for it. Give me everything you've got for the next two hundred yards and let's do it!" and he started to sprint to the finish line. Abbie followed him. She moaned and groaned for those last few yards, but she stayed with her daddy every step. As they finally crossed the finish line, Abbie fell to her knees and gasped for air as her daddy stopped the watch.

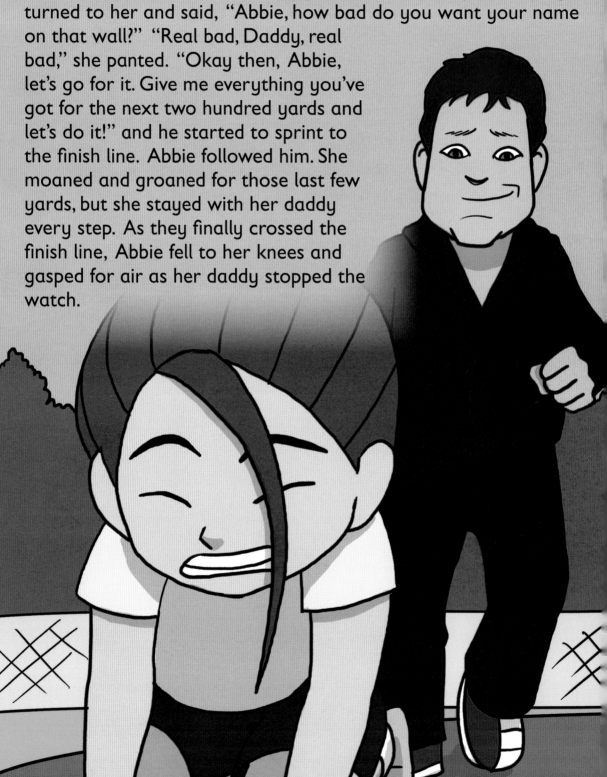

He stood staring at the watch, "Oh my, Abbie!" he said, shaking his head. She looked up at him and gasped, "What Daddy, what?" "Abbie, you're not going to believe what you just did," he said. She jumped up and grabbed his hand, "What, Daddy, what did I do?" He wrapped his arm around her shoulder and showed Abbie the stop watch. "Abbie, you just ran that mile in seven minutes and fifty-four seconds! You beat your goal by over two and a half minutes!" he cheered as he gave Abbie a big bear hug. Abbie grabbed the watch. "Oh my gosh, Daddy, oh my gosh," she screamed. "Daddy, I can't believe it! Is this right, did I really run a mile in under eight minutes?" She jumped up and down while staring at the watch. "Yes, Abbie, it's right. And not only that, you beat the challenge goal by over a minute!" He swung her around and laughed, "Abbie, you were great out there...you were hurting and wanted to quit, but you stayed with it, ran hard and look what you've done!

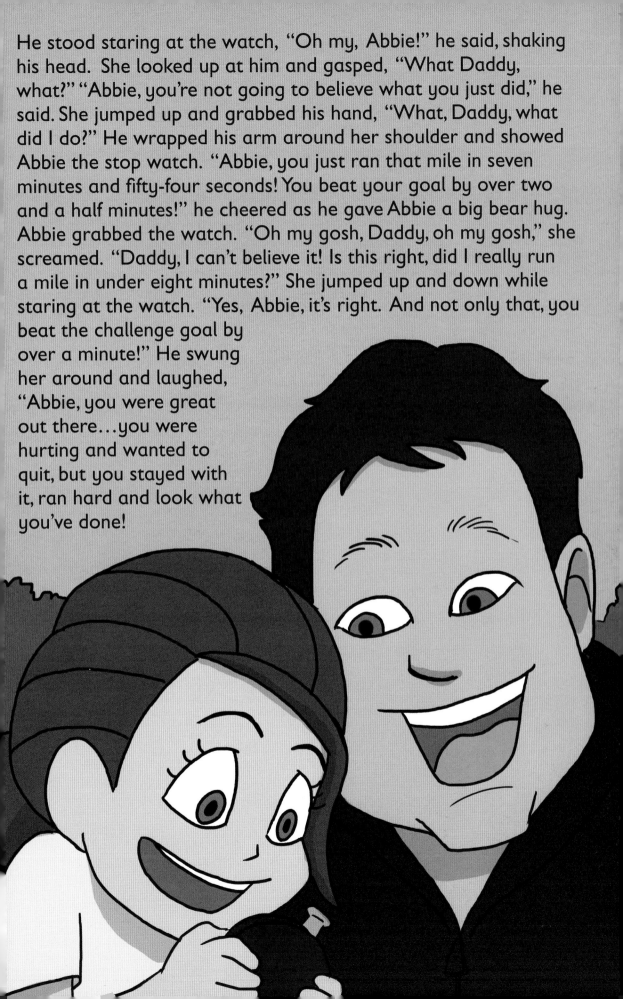

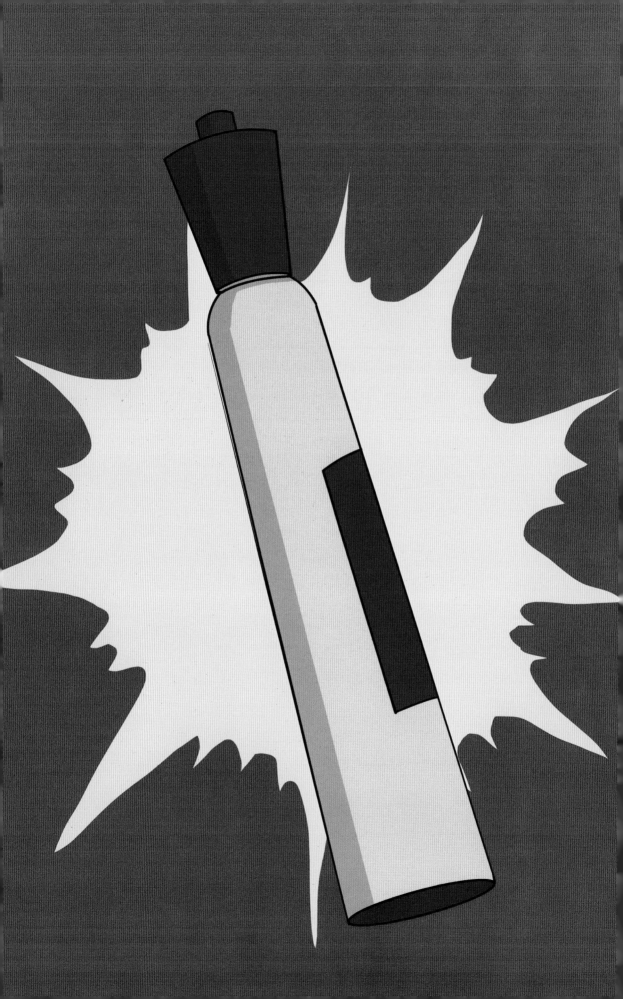

You not only reached your goal, but you beat it by a lot." He held her for a moment and then stepped back, "You know what this means don't you?" he asked her. "No, Daddy, what does it mean?" she shrugged. Her daddy reached into his pocket, slowly pulled out the largest blue marker Abbie had ever seen and handed it to her. "It means that you're going to need this after you take your fitness test next week!" Her face lit up, she screeched in delight, and snatched the marker from his hand. "Oh, Daddy, thank you, thank you, thank you! We did it, we did it!" Abbie wept with joy and wrapped her arms around him, rocking him side to side. He stepped back again, put his hands on her shoulders and stared into her teary eyes, "No, Abbie," he answered her, "you did it, Abbie…you did it!"

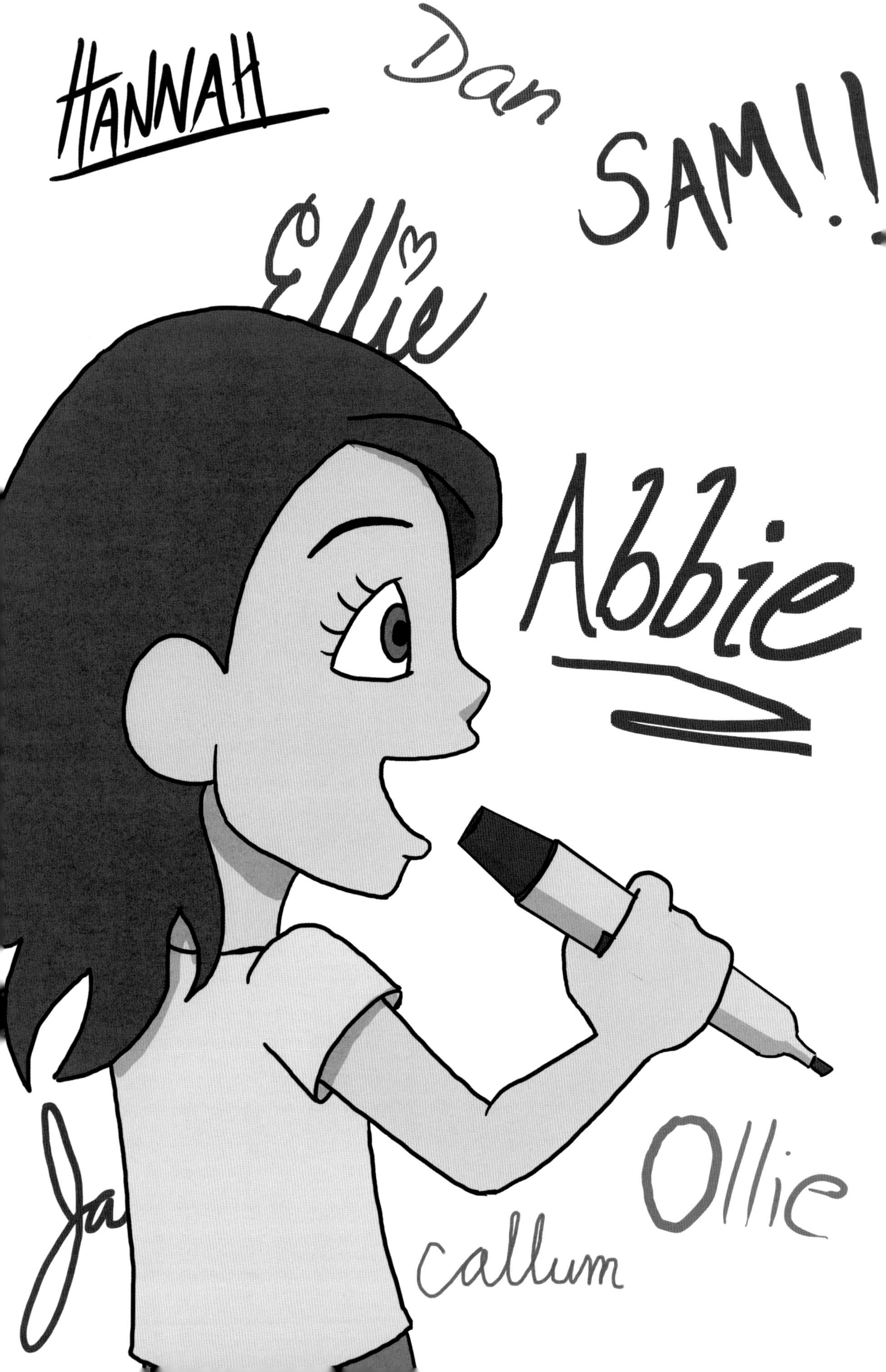

The next week Abbie took her second fitness test of the school year. She beat the challenge goals in curl ups, push-ups, sit and reach, and the mile. In just six months of daily exercise, Abbie had progressed from a very unfit child to one of the fittest in her class. Using that big blue marker, it was with great pride and a huge smile that Abbie finally put her name up on that wall.

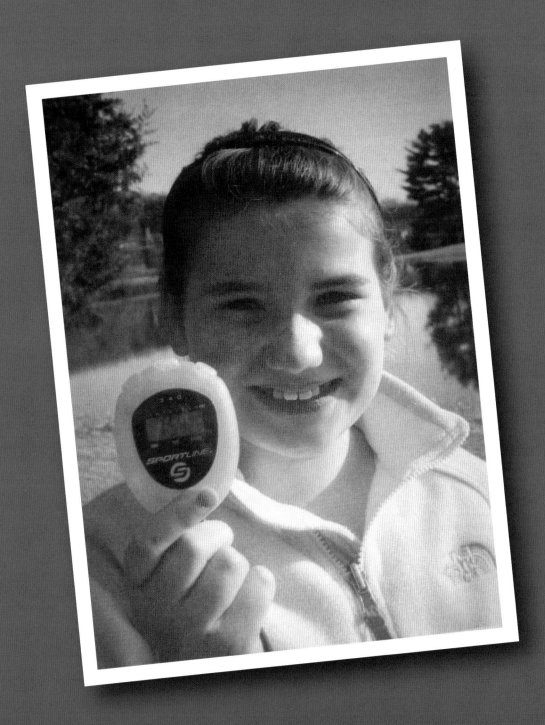

I hope that you have enjoyed my story. I am now 13 years old and in the seventh grade. I still don't like sports much and I still prefer to 'hang out' instead of 'work out,' but I do go for a brisk walk with my mom or dad at least one hour every day and I do my curl ups and push-ups every night. In my most recent fitness test at school, I beat all four fitness goals again, including 75 curl-ups in 3 minutes against a goal of 52.

While getting fit, I also started learning more about proper eating habits and nutrition. This helped me a lot. For example, did you know that a normal 'bowl of cereal' at breakfast can be as much as 750 calories? I now eat just 1 ¼ cups of cereal every day, which is only 250 calories. That is 3,500 calories less per week. Guess how many calories are in one pound of body fat…3,500 calories! So that is a very big difference. My favorite nutrition books are the *Eat This Not That* series, but there are lots of other very good books on nutrition too. Just be sure to find at least one that you like.

When I wasn't fit, I didn't like doing a lot of fun stuff with my family. Now, I love to swim, play tennis and go on long bike rides and hikes with my mom, dad and brother. When I wasn't fit, I didn't have much energy for studying or doing my homework. Now, I am an honor roll student and getting As and Bs in school. Getting fit was the best thing I have ever done. I hope that this book will help you to get fit too. It's all up to you, you can do it!

Yours in fitness,
Abbie Werner

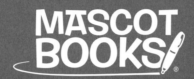